Sleep Paralysis

All You Need To Know

Josh C. Pete

Table Of Contents

1. Introduction

- 1.1 Definition of Sleep Paralysis

Sleep paralysis is a temporary inability to move or speak that occurs when transitioning between sleep stages or upon waking up. During episodes of sleep paralysis, individuals may experience a sense of being awake but unable to move, often accompanied by hallucinations and a feeling of pressure on the chest. This phenomenon typically occurs during the rapid eye movement (REM) stage of sleep when dreaming takes place, due to a temporary disruption in the normal muscle atonia that accompanies REM sleep. Sleep paralysis can be a distressing experience, but it is usually harmless and tends to resolve on its own within a few seconds to minutes.

- 1.2 Historical Background

The historical background of sleep paralysis is rich and varied, with mentions dating back centuries across different cultures and civilizations. Here are some key points in the historical timeline of sleep paralysis:

1. **Ancient Cultures:** References to sleep paralysis can be found in ancient texts and folklore from various civilizations, including the Greeks, Romans, Egyptians, and Chinese. These accounts often described the experience as being visited by supernatural entities or spirits during sleep.

2. **Medieval Europe:** During the Middle Ages, sleep paralysis was commonly associated with beliefs in witchcraft and demonic possession. It was often interpreted as evidence of nocturnal attacks by malevolent spirits or witches,

leading to fear and superstition surrounding the condition.

3. Scientific Exploration: The scientific study of sleep paralysis began to emerge in the 19th century with the development of psychology and sleep medicine. Researchers started to investigate the physiological mechanisms underlying the phenomenon and distinguish it from supernatural explanations.

4. Psychological Theories: In the early 20th century, psychoanalytic theories proposed by Sigmund Freud and others suggested that sleep paralysis was linked to repressed anxieties and unconscious conflicts. This perspective contributed to a more nuanced understanding of the psychological aspects of the experience.

5. Cross-Cultural Perspectives: Anthropological studies have highlighted the cultural variations in how sleep paralysis is interpreted and experienced around the world. While some cultures continue to view it through supernatural lenses, others approach it from a more medical or psychological standpoint.

6. Contemporary Research: In recent decades, advancements in sleep science and neurology have deepened our understanding of sleep paralysis. Studies have identified the role of REM sleep dysfunction and disruptions in the sleep-wake cycle in predisposing individuals to sleep paralysis episodes.

Overall, the historical background of sleep paralysis reflects a complex interplay between cultural beliefs, scientific inquiry, and psychological interpretations over time. This multifaceted perspective underscores the importance of considering both cultural context and scientific evidence in understanding and addressing sleep paralysis.

- 1.3 Prevalence and Occurrence

The prevalence and occurrence of sleep paralysis vary across populations and are influenced by various factors such as age, gender, and cultural background. Here are some key points regarding the prevalence and occurrence of sleep paralysis:

1. **Overall Prevalence:** Sleep paralysis is relatively common, with studies suggesting that a significant portion of the population will experience at least one episode in their lifetime. Estimates of prevalence vary, but research indicates that anywhere from 5% to 60% of individuals may experience sleep paralysis at some point.

2. **Age and Gender:** Sleep paralysis can occur at any age but tends to be most prevalent in young adults,

particularly those in their twenties and thirties. There is some evidence to suggest that women may be slightly more likely to experience sleep paralysis than men, although findings have been inconsistent across studies.

3. Cultural Factors: The prevalence of sleep paralysis can vary significantly across different cultural and ethnic groups. Cultural beliefs and practices surrounding sleep, dreams, and spirituality may influence how sleep paralysis is perceived and experienced within a particular community.

4. Association with Sleep Disorders: Sleep paralysis is often associated with other sleep disorders, particularly narcolepsy. Research has shown that individuals with narcolepsy, a neurological disorder characterized by excessive daytime sleepiness and disrupted REM sleep, are more likely to experience sleep paralysis.

5. Stress and Sleep Deprivation: Episodes of sleep paralysis have been linked to periods of increased stress, anxiety, and sleep deprivation. Stressful life events, irregular sleep schedules, and disrupted sleep patterns can all contribute to the occurrence of sleep paralysis episodes.

6. Family History and Genetics: There is some evidence to suggest that genetic factors may play a role in predisposing individuals to sleep paralysis. Family history studies have found that relatives of individuals with narcolepsy and other sleep disorders may be more likely to experience sleep paralysis themselves.

7. Lifetime Frequency: For most individuals, sleep paralysis is an infrequent occurrence, with episodes occurring sporadically throughout their lives. However, some individuals may experience recurrent or even frequent episodes of sleep paralysis, which can have a significant impact on their sleep quality and overall well-being.

Overall, the prevalence and occurrence of sleep paralysis are influenced by a complex interplay of biological, psychological, and environmental factors. Further research is needed to better understand the underlying mechanisms and to develop effective strategies for prevention and management.

2. The Physiology of Sleep

- 2.1 Stages of Sleep

The stages of sleep are typically divided into non-REM (rapid eye movement) sleep and REM sleep. Each stage serves a different purpose and is characterized by distinct patterns of brain activity and physiological changes. Here's an overview of the stages of sleep:

1. Wakefulness:
   - This is the state when you are fully awake and alert. Brain activity is characterized by beta waves, and muscle tone is active.

2. Non-REM Sleep:
   Non-REM sleep is further divided into three stages: N1, N2, and N3.

a. Stage N1 (Transition to Sleep):

- This is the lightest stage of sleep, occurring as you transition from wakefulness to sleep.

- Brain activity begins to slow down, and you may experience drifting thoughts or brief muscle twitches.

- It's easy to be awakened from this stage.

b. Stage N2 (Light Sleep):

- Stage N2 is characterized by a decrease in heart rate and body temperature.

- Brain waves become slower with occasional bursts of rapid activity known as sleep spindles.

- This stage makes up the majority of sleep time in a typical night's sleep.

c. Stage N3 (Deep Sleep or Slow-Wave Sleep):

- Deep sleep is the stage where the body undergoes restorative processes, such as tissue repair and growth.

- Brain waves slow down even further, with the presence of slow delta waves.

- It can be difficult to wake someone from this stage, and if awakened, they may feel groggy or disoriented.

3. REM Sleep (Rapid Eye Movement Sleep):

- REM sleep is characterized by rapid eye movements, increased brain activity, and muscle paralysis (atonia).

- This stage is when most dreaming occurs, and it's associated with emotional processing and memory consolidation.

- Physiological changes include increased heart rate, irregular breathing, and temporary paralysis of voluntary muscles.

- REM sleep cycles typically occur in intervals of about 90 minutes throughout the night, becoming longer and more frequent toward morning.

The sleep cycle progresses through these stages multiple times during the night, with each cycle lasting approximately 90 to 120 minutes. As the night progresses, the proportion of time spent in REM sleep increases, while the amount of deep sleep decreases. This cycling between non-REM and REM sleep stages is essential for overall sleep quality and restoration.

- 2.2 REM Sleep and Muscle Atonia

REM (Rapid Eye Movement) sleep is a stage of sleep characterized by rapid eye movements, vivid dreaming, and heightened brain activity. One of the key features of REM sleep is muscle atonia, which refers to a temporary paralysis of voluntary muscles throughout the body. Here's more detail about REM sleep and muscle atonia:

1. REM Sleep Characteristics:

- REM sleep typically occurs cyclically throughout the night, with each cycle lasting approximately 90 to 120 minutes.

- It is associated with increased brain activity, similar to wakefulness, as evidenced by EEG (electroencephalogram) recordings showing beta and gamma waves.

- During REM sleep, the brain becomes highly active, while the body remains largely immobile due to muscle atonia.

2. Muscle Atonia:

- Muscle atonia refers to the state of muscle paralysis or lack of muscle tone that occurs during REM sleep.

- This paralysis affects most voluntary muscles in the body, including those in the limbs and trunk, but excludes certain muscles essential for vital functions such as respiration and eye movements.

- Muscle atonia is thought to be mediated by the inhibition of motor neurons in the spinal cord during REM sleep, preventing the execution of voluntary movements.

3. Purpose of Muscle Atonia:
- Muscle atonia serves several important functions during REM sleep:
- Prevents individuals from physically acting out their dreams, which could result in injury to themselves or others.
- Facilitates the vividness and immersion of dreams by preventing the body from responding to dream content.
- Supports the consolidation of memories and emotional processing associated with dreaming by maintaining a dissociation between the brain's activity and physical movements.

4. Disruption of Muscle Atonia:
- Disorders or disruptions in muscle atonia during REM sleep can lead to various phenomena, such as REM sleep behavior disorder (RBD).
- In RBD, individuals physically act out their dreams, often with violent or

vigorous movements, due to a lack of muscle paralysis.

- Other sleep disorders, such as sleep paralysis, can also involve disruptions in the normal transition between REM sleep and wakefulness, leading to temporary muscle atonia while awake.

Overall, muscle atonia during REM sleep is a vital mechanism that ensures the safety and integrity of sleep by preventing the body from acting out dreams while allowing the brain to engage in vivid and immersive dream experiences.

- 2.3 Sleep Disorders Overview

An overview of sleep disorders encompasses a wide range of conditions that affect the quality, timing, and duration of sleep. These disorders can disrupt sleep patterns and have significant impacts on overall health, well-being, and daily functioning. Here's an overview of some common sleep disorders:

1. Insomnia:
- Insomnia involves difficulty falling asleep, staying asleep, or waking up too early and not being able to fall back asleep.
- It can be acute (short-term) or chronic (long-term) and may be caused by various factors, including stress, anxiety, depression, medications, or medical conditions.

2. Obstructive Sleep Apnea (OSA):
- OSA is a sleep-related breathing disorder characterized by repetitive episodes of complete or partial obstruction of the upper airway during sleep.
- It leads to disrupted breathing patterns, loud snoring, and fragmented sleep, often resulting in excessive daytime sleepiness, fatigue, and other health complications.

3. Central Sleep Apnea (CSA):

- CSA occurs when the brain fails to send the appropriate signals to the muscles that control breathing during sleep.

- Unlike OSA, which is caused by physical obstruction of the airway, CSA is characterized by pauses in breathing without associated airway obstruction.

4. Sleep-Related Movement Disorders:

- Restless Legs Syndrome (RLS) is a movement disorder characterized by uncomfortable sensations in the legs and an irresistible urge to move them, often disrupting sleep.

- Periodic Limb Movement Disorder (PLMD) involves repetitive limb movements during sleep, leading to frequent awakenings and poor sleep quality.

5. Parasomnias:

- Parasomnias are abnormal behaviors or experiences that occur during sleep or during transitions between sleep stages.

- Examples include sleepwalking, sleep talking, confusional arousals, nightmares, and night terrors.

6. Hypersomnias:

- Hypersomnias are conditions characterized by excessive daytime sleepiness and difficulty staying awake during the day, despite getting enough sleep at night.

- Conditions such as narcolepsy and idiopathic hypersomnia fall into this category.

7. Circadian Rhythm Sleep-Wake Disorders:

- These disorders involve disruptions in the timing of sleep and wakefulness, often due to abnormalities in the body's internal circadian clock.

- Examples include delayed sleep phase disorder, advanced sleep phase disorder, and shift work sleep disorder.

8. Sleep-Related Hypoventilation Disorders:

- These disorders are characterized by abnormal breathing patterns during sleep, resulting in decreased oxygen levels and increased carbon dioxide levels in the blood.
- Conditions such as obesity hypoventilation syndrome fall into this category.

9. Sleep Disorders Associated with Other Medical or Psychiatric Conditions:

- Certain medical or psychiatric conditions can also impact sleep, either directly or indirectly. Examples include mood disorders, anxiety disorders, neurodegenerative diseases, and chronic pain conditions.

10. Other Sleep Disorders:

- This category includes less common or emerging sleep disorders, such as sleep-related eating disorders, sleep-related groaning, and sleep-related hallucinations.

Managing and treating sleep disorders often requires a multidisciplinary approach involving healthcare professionals such as sleep specialists, pulmonologists, neurologists, psychologists, and other specialists. Treatment options may include lifestyle modifications, behavioral therapies, medications, and interventions such as continuous positive airway pressure (CPAP) therapy for sleep apnea.

3. Understanding Sleep Paralysis

- *3.1 Definition and Characteristics*

Understanding sleep paralysis involves exploring its definition, characteristics, underlying mechanisms, contributing factors, and potential implications. Here's an overview:

1. Definition and Characteristics:
- Sleep paralysis is a temporary inability to move or speak that occurs during transitions between sleep stages or upon waking up.
- During episodes of sleep paralysis, individuals may experience a sense of being awake but unable to move, often accompanied by hallucinations and a feeling of pressure on the chest.
- These episodes can be distressing and may lead to feelings of fear, panic, or helplessness.

2. Symptoms and Experiences:

-    Common symptoms of sleep paralysis include the inability to move or speak, sensations of pressure or weight on the chest, and visual or auditory hallucinations.

- Hallucinations during sleep paralysis may take various forms, such as seeing shadowy figures, feeling a presence in the room, or hearing strange noises or voices.

-    Individuals experiencing sleep paralysis may feel a sense of terror or impending doom, but these feelings typically dissipate once the episode ends.

3. Factors Contributing to Sleep Paralysis:

- Sleep paralysis can be influenced by various factors, including genetics, sleep deprivation, irregular sleep schedules, stress, anxiety, and other sleep disorders.

- Genetic predisposition may play a role in some cases, as individuals with a family history of sleep disorders may be more likely to experience sleep paralysis.

- Sleep paralysis often occurs during the rapid eye movement (REM) stage of sleep, when dreaming takes place, and is thought to result from a temporary disruption in the normal muscle atonia that accompanies REM sleep.

4. Implications and Management:

- While sleep paralysis episodes are generally harmless and tend to resolve on their own within a few seconds to minutes, they can have significant implications for sleep quality, mental health, and overall well-being.

- Coping strategies during episodes may include focusing on controlled breathing, attempting to move smaller muscles like the fingers or toes, or trying to wake oneself up fully.

- Managing contributing factors such as stress, improving sleep hygiene, and seeking treatment for underlying sleep disorders may help reduce the frequency or severity of sleep paralysis episodes.

Understanding sleep paralysis involves recognizing its complex interplay of physiological, psychological, and environmental factors, as well as its potential impact on individuals' lives. Continued research into the mechanisms and management of sleep paralysis is essential for providing support and guidance to those who experience this phenomenon.

- 3.2 Types of Sleep Paralysis

Sleep paralysis can be classified into two main types: isolated sleep paralysis and recurrent isolated sleep paralysis.

1. Isolated Sleep Paralysis:

- Isolated sleep paralysis refers to occasional episodes that occur infrequently and are not associated with any underlying sleep disorder.

- Individuals experiencing isolated sleep paralysis may have one or a few episodes throughout their lifetime, typically occurring during periods of heightened stress, sleep deprivation, or changes in sleep patterns.

- Isolated sleep paralysis episodes may be frightening or distressing, but they are generally harmless and tend to resolve on their own within a few seconds to minutes.

- This type of sleep paralysis is often not indicative of a chronic sleep disorder and may occur in otherwise healthy individuals.

2. Recurrent Isolated Sleep Paralysis:

- Recurrent isolated sleep paralysis involves recurrent episodes of sleep paralysis that may occur multiple times over an individual's lifetime.

- These episodes are typically similar in duration, frequency, and associated symptoms, and they may follow a pattern of occurring during specific periods or under certain conditions.

- While recurrent isolated sleep paralysis shares similarities with isolated sleep paralysis in terms of symptoms and characteristics, it differs in terms of frequency and predictability.

- Individuals experiencing recurrent isolated sleep paralysis may find the episodes distressing or disruptive to their sleep, leading to increased anxiety or fear surrounding sleep.

It's important to note that while isolated sleep paralysis and recurrent isolated sleep paralysis are the two main types often discussed in the literature, sleep paralysis can also occur as a symptom of other sleep disorders, such as narcolepsy. In these cases, sleep paralysis may be accompanied by other symptoms such as excessive daytime sleepiness, cataplexy (sudden loss of muscle tone), hypnagogic hallucinations (hallucinations when falling asleep), or disrupted nighttime sleep. Identifying the underlying cause of sleep paralysis is crucial for appropriate management and treatment.

- 3.3 Symptoms and Experiences

The symptoms and experiences of sleep paralysis can vary from person to person, but they typically involve a combination of physical sensations, perceptual distortions, and emotional responses. Here are some common symptoms and experiences associated with sleep paralysis:

1. Inability to Move or Speak:

- The hallmark symptom of sleep paralysis is the temporary inability to move or speak, despite being consciously aware of one's surroundings.

- Individuals may feel as though their muscles are paralyzed or locked in place, making it impossible to perform voluntary movements or vocalize.

2. Sensations of Pressure or Weight:

- Many people report feeling a sensation of pressure or weight on their chest during sleep paralysis episodes.

- This sensation can range from mild discomfort to a feeling of suffocation or being crushed, contributing to feelings of fear or panic.

3. Visual and Auditory Hallucinations:

- Sleep paralysis often involves vivid hallucinations that can manifest as visual, auditory, or tactile sensations.

- Visual hallucinations may include seeing shadowy figures, strange shapes, or distorted images in the environment.

- Auditory hallucinations may involve hearing voices, whispers, or other sounds that seem to come from within the room or from outside sources.

- Tactile hallucinations, such as feeling a presence in the room or sensing someone touching or grabbing you, are also common.

4. Feelings of Fear or Panic:

- Sleep paralysis episodes are frequently accompanied by intense feelings of fear, panic, or impending doom.

- These emotional responses may be triggered by the sensation of paralysis, hallucinations, or a sense of vulnerability associated with being unable to move or defend oneself.

5. Sense of Time Distortion:

- Many individuals report a distorted sense of time during sleep paralysis, with episodes often feeling much longer than they actually are.

- Time may seem to stretch or slow down, leading to a subjective experience of the episode lasting for an extended period.

6. Difficulty Breathing:

- Some individuals may experience sensations of difficulty breathing or suffocation during sleep paralysis episodes.
- While this sensation is typically a result of the perceived pressure on the chest or the sense of paralysis, it can contribute to feelings of anxiety or distress.

7. Awareness of Surroundings:

- Despite being unable to move or speak, individuals experiencing sleep paralysis are usually fully conscious and aware of their surroundings.
- They may be able to perceive sounds, sights, and sensations in the

environment, adding to the overall intensity of the experience.

Overall, the symptoms and experiences of sleep paralysis can be highly distressing and frightening for those who experience them. While episodes are typically brief and resolve on their own, they can have a significant impact on sleep quality, mental health, and overall well-being. Developing coping strategies and seeking support from healthcare professionals can help individuals manage and reduce the frequency or severity of sleep paralysis episodes.

- *3.4 Factors Contributing to Sleep Paralysis*

Several factors can contribute to the occurrence of sleep paralysis, including biological, psychological, and environmental influences. Here are some key factors that may contribute to sleep paralysis:

1. Genetics and Family History:

- There is evidence to suggest that genetic factors may predispose individuals to sleep paralysis. Family history studies have shown that relatives of individuals with sleep disorders, such as narcolepsy, may be more likely to experience sleep paralysis themselves.

2. Disrupted Sleep Patterns:

- Irregular sleep schedules, frequent disruptions to sleep, and poor sleep hygiene can increase the likelihood of experiencing sleep paralysis.

- Sleep deprivation, whether chronic or acute, can disrupt the normal sleep-wake cycle and increase the risk of sleep paralysis episodes.

3. Stress and Anxiety:

- Stressful life events, anxiety, and emotional distress can exacerbate sleep disturbances and contribute to the occurrence of sleep paralysis.

- Individuals who experience high levels of stress or anxiety may be more susceptible to sleep paralysis episodes, particularly during periods of heightened emotional arousal.

4. Sleep Disorders:

- Certain sleep disorders, such as narcolepsy, insomnia, and obstructive sleep apnea, are associated with an increased risk of sleep paralysis.

- In narcolepsy, which involves disruptions to the normal sleep-wake cycle, sleep paralysis is a common symptom experienced during transitions between wakefulness and REM sleep.

5. Medications and Substance Use:

- Certain medications, such as antidepressants, stimulants, and drugs that affect neurotransmitter levels in the brain, may influence sleep architecture and increase the likelihood of sleep paralysis.

- Substance use, including alcohol, nicotine, and recreational drugs, can also disrupt sleep patterns and contribute to sleep paralysis episodes.

6. Sleep Position and Environment:

- Sleeping in supine (on the back) positions may increase the risk of experiencing sleep paralysis, as this position is associated with a higher incidence of obstructive sleep apnea and disrupted breathing patterns.

- Environmental factors, such as noise, light, temperature, and comfort level, can also impact sleep quality and contribute to sleep paralysis episodes.

7. Psychological Factors:

- Psychological factors, such as personality traits, coping mechanisms, and cognitive processes, may influence susceptibility to sleep paralysis.

- Individuals who are prone to dissociative experiences, hypnagogic hallucinations, or altered states of consciousness may be more likely to experience sleep paralysis.

8. Cultural and Sociocultural Influences:

- Cultural beliefs, superstitions, and narratives surrounding sleep and dreams may shape individuals' perceptions and experiences of sleep paralysis.

- Sociocultural factors, such as socioeconomic status, cultural norms, and access to healthcare resources, can also impact sleep quality and contribute to sleep paralysis risk.

Overall, sleep paralysis is a multifaceted phenomenon influenced by a combination of biological, psychological, and environmental factors. Understanding these contributing factors can help individuals and healthcare professionals identify strategies for managing and reducing the frequency or severity of sleep paralysis episodes.

4. Cultural and Historical Perspectives

- 4.1 Sleep Paralysis in Folklore and Mythology

Sleep paralysis has been a subject of fascination and interpretation in folklore and mythology across various cultures throughout history. Here's how sleep paralysis has been perceived and depicted in folklore and mythology:

1. Europe:

- In European folklore, sleep paralysis has often been associated with supernatural entities such as witches, demons, or malevolent spirits.

- Tales of the "night hag" or "old hag syndrome" describe a demonic entity that sits on the chest of sleeping individuals, causing feelings of pressure and suffocation associated with sleep paralysis.

- Beliefs in witchcraft and sorcery led to the attribution of sleep paralysis episodes to nocturnal visits by witches or evil spirits, resulting in fear and superstition surrounding the phenomenon.

2. Africa:

- In some African cultures, sleep paralysis is interpreted as the work of malevolent spirits or witchcraft.

- It is believed that witches or evil spirits can enter a person's body while they sleep, causing paralysis and disturbing dreams.

- Rituals and protective measures, such as amulets or charms, may be used to ward off evil spirits and prevent sleep paralysis.

3. Asia:

- Across various Asian cultures, sleep paralysis is often associated with supernatural beings or entities.

- In Japanese folklore, sleep paralysis is known as "kanashibari" or "kagome, kagome," and is attributed to the actions of malevolent spirits or ghosts.

- Similar beliefs are found in other Asian cultures, where sleep paralysis may be interpreted as an encounter with ghosts, demons, or ancestral spirits.

4. Americas:

- Indigenous cultures in the Americas have their own interpretations of sleep paralysis, often linking it to spiritual beliefs and shamanic practices.

- In some Native American traditions, sleep paralysis may be seen as a form of spiritual initiation or communication with the spirit world.

- Stories and legends passed down through generations may incorporate sleep paralysis as a theme, illustrating its significance in cultural narratives.

5. Middle East:

- In Middle Eastern folklore, sleep paralysis may be attributed to the influence of jinn, supernatural beings mentioned in Islamic mythology.

- It is believed that jinn can interact with humans in various ways, including causing sleep disturbances and paralysis.

- Protective rituals and prayers are often used to ward off jinn and prevent sleep paralysis episodes.

Overall, sleep paralysis has been woven into the fabric of cultural beliefs, superstitions, and mythologies around the world, reflecting humanity's attempts to make sense of this mysterious and often frightening phenomenon. While modern science offers explanations rooted in neurobiology and sleep medicine, the cultural interpretations of sleep paralysis continue to shape individuals' perceptions and experiences of the phenomenon.

Sleep paralysis has long been a source of inspiration for artists and writers, influencing various forms of art and literature throughout history. Here's how sleep paralysis has influenced art and literature:

1. Visual Art:

- Sleep paralysis and its associated hallucinations have been depicted in visual art, ranging from paintings and drawings to sculptures and illustrations.

- Artists often portray the surreal and unsettling aspects of sleep paralysis, capturing the feeling of being trapped between wakefulness and dreaming.

- Visual representations may include images of shadowy figures, distorted faces, or surreal landscapes that evoke the eerie and disorienting nature of sleep paralysis.

2. Literature:

- Sleep paralysis has been a recurring theme in literature, appearing in various works of fiction, poetry, and non-fiction writing.

- Authors explore the psychological and existential implications of sleep paralysis, delving into themes of fear, mortality, and the supernatural.

- Sleep paralysis is often used as a narrative device to create tension, suspense, or psychological depth in storytelling.

- Some authors draw from personal experiences of sleep paralysis to craft vivid and immersive descriptions that resonate with readers who have had similar experiences.

3. Symbolism and Metaphor:

- Sleep paralysis is sometimes used as a metaphor or symbolic motif in art and literature to represent broader themes of powerlessness, oppression, or existential dread.

- It may symbolize the feeling of being trapped in one's own mind or the struggle to break free from psychological or emotional constraints.

- Sleep paralysis can also serve as a metaphor for the liminal space between consciousness and unconsciousness, reality and illusion, or life and death.

4. Cultural and Folklore References:

- Art and literature often draw upon cultural beliefs, folklore, and mythology surrounding sleep paralysis to enrich storytelling and imagery.

- References to supernatural entities, spiritual experiences, or cultural rituals associated with sleep paralysis may add depth and resonance to artistic interpretations.

- Artists and writers may incorporate elements of cultural symbolism and storytelling to explore the cultural significance of sleep paralysis within specific communities or traditions.

5. Exploration of Consciousness and Perception:
   - Sleep paralysis offers fertile ground for exploring themes related to consciousness, perception, and the nature of reality.
   - Artists and writers may use sleep paralysis as a lens through which to examine the boundaries between waking life and the dream world, exploring the shifting landscapes of the mind and the mysteries of human consciousness.

Overall, sleep paralysis has left its mark on art and literature, inspiring creators to explore themes of fear, spirituality, and the human condition. Through visual imagery, narrative storytelling, and metaphorical expression, artists and writers continue to grapple with the enigmatic nature of sleep paralysis and its profound impact on the human psyche.

5. Theories and Explanations

- 5.1 Neurological Explanations

Neurological explanations for sleep paralysis focus on the underlying brain mechanisms and physiological processes that contribute to its occurrence. Here are some key neurological explanations for sleep paralysis:

1. REM Sleep Dysfunction:

- Sleep paralysis is closely associated with rapid eye movement (REM) sleep, a stage of sleep characterized by vivid dreaming, rapid eye movements, and muscle atonia (temporary paralysis of voluntary muscles).

- During REM sleep, the brainstem inhibits the activity of motor neurons in the spinal cord, leading to muscle atonia and preventing individuals from physically acting out their dreams.

- In sleep paralysis, disruptions in the normal transition between REM sleep and wakefulness can result in the persistence of muscle atonia upon waking up, leading to the sensation of being unable to move or speak.

2. REM Rebound:

- REM rebound refers to an increase in the duration and intensity of REM sleep following periods of sleep deprivation or disrupted sleep.

- Sleep deprivation, irregular sleep schedules, or disturbances in sleep architecture can lead to REM rebound, increasing the likelihood of experiencing sleep paralysis episodes.

- The rebound effect may result in more frequent or intense REM sleep, leading to disruptions in the normal regulation of muscle tone and sleep-wake transitions.

3. Dysfunction in Brainstem and Thalamus:

- Neuroimaging studies have identified abnormalities in brain regions involved in regulating sleep and wakefulness, including the brainstem and thalamus, in individuals with sleep paralysis.

- Dysfunction in the brainstem, which plays a key role in coordinating sleep cycles and controlling muscle activity during sleep, may contribute to disruptions in REM sleep and the persistence of muscle atonia.

- Alterations in thalamic function, which is involved in sensory processing and consciousness, may also influence the perception of sensory experiences and hallucinations during sleep paralysis.

4. Hyperarousal and Altered Consciousness:

- Some researchers propose that sleep paralysis may involve a state of heightened arousal or altered consciousness, characterized by increased activity in brain regions associated with wakefulness and vigilance.

- This hyperarousal state may lead to an amplification of sensory perceptions, hallucinations, and emotional responses during sleep paralysis episodes.

- Changes in neurotransmitter levels, such as serotonin and dopamine, may also play a role in modulating arousal and regulating REM sleep, contributing to the occurrence of sleep paralysis.

5. Genetic and Environmental Factors:

- Genetic predisposition may influence susceptibility to sleep paralysis, with some individuals showing a familial or hereditary tendency to experience sleep disturbances or REM sleep abnormalities.

- Environmental factors, such as stress, anxiety, and sleep disturbances, can interact with genetic factors to increase the risk of sleep paralysis episodes.

   - Gene-environment interactions may influence the expression of sleep-related genes and the functioning of neural circuits involved in sleep regulation and motor control.

Overall, neurological explanations for sleep paralysis emphasize the complex interplay of brain regions, neurotransmitter systems, and genetic and environmental factors in contributing to this phenomenon. Further research is needed to elucidate the underlying mechanisms and develop targeted interventions for managing and preventing sleep paralysis.

- 5.2 Psychological Explanations

Psychological explanations for sleep paralysis focus on the role of psychological factors, beliefs, and experiences in influencing the occurrence and interpretation of sleep paralysis episodes. Here are some key psychological explanations for sleep paralysis:

1. Stress and Anxiety:

- Stressful life events, anxiety, and emotional distress can contribute to the occurrence of sleep paralysis episodes.

- Heightened levels of stress or anxiety may disrupt sleep patterns, leading to disturbances in REM sleep and an increased risk of experiencing sleep paralysis.

- Individuals who are prone to anxiety or who experience high levels of stress may be more susceptible to sleep paralysis, particularly during periods of heightened emotional arousal.

2. Cognitive Factors:

- Cognitive factors, such as beliefs, expectations, and cognitive biases, can influence the interpretation and experience of sleep paralysis.

- Individuals who hold beliefs or cultural narratives associating sleep paralysis with supernatural entities or malevolent spirits may interpret their experiences in line with these beliefs, leading to feelings of fear or panic.

- Cognitive biases, such as attentional biases or memory distortions, may also shape the perception of sensory experiences and hallucinations during sleep paralysis episodes.

3. Sleep-Related Beliefs and Experiences:

- Previous experiences with sleep disturbances, nightmares, or altered states of consciousness can influence susceptibility to sleep paralysis.

- Individuals who have experienced traumatic or unsettling sleep-related experiences may be more likely to interpret sleep paralysis episodes as threatening or distressing.

- Beliefs about sleep, dreams, and the nature of consciousness can also influence how individuals perceive and interpret their experiences during sleep paralysis.

4. Cultural and Sociocultural Influences:

- Cultural beliefs, superstitions, and social norms surrounding sleep and dreams can shape individuals' interpretations of sleep paralysis.

- Cultural narratives and folklore may provide frameworks for understanding and contextualizing sleep paralysis experiences, influencing emotional responses and coping strategies.

- Sociocultural factors, such as socioeconomic status, access to healthcare resources, and exposure to media representations of sleep paralysis, can also impact individuals' perceptions and experiences of the phenomenon.

5. Emotional Regulation and Coping Mechanisms:

- Individual differences in emotional regulation and coping strategies may influence how individuals respond to sleep paralysis episodes.

- Effective coping mechanisms, such as relaxation techniques, cognitive reframing, and social support, can help mitigate feelings of fear or distress associated with sleep paralysis.

- Conversely, maladaptive coping strategies, such as avoidance or rumination, may exacerbate feelings of anxiety or helplessness during sleep paralysis episodes.

Overall, psychological explanations for sleep paralysis highlight the complex interplay of psychological, cognitive, and sociocultural factors in shaping individuals' experiences and responses to this phenomenon. Understanding these psychological factors can inform interventions aimed at reducing the frequency or severity of sleep paralysis episodes and improving overall well-being.

- *5.3 Parapsychological and Supernatural Interpretations*

Parapsychological and supernatural interpretations of sleep paralysis delve into the realm of the paranormal, exploring the possibility of otherworldly or supernatural explanations for the phenomenon. Here are some perspectives from parapsychology and supernatural beliefs regarding sleep paralysis:

1. Influence of Malevolent Entities:

- Many cultures and belief systems attribute sleep paralysis to the influence of malevolent entities, such as demons, spirits, or supernatural beings.

- According to these interpretations, sleep paralysis may occur when individuals are vulnerable to spiritual intrusion or attack during periods of sleep or altered states of consciousness.

- Some cultures refer to sleep paralysis as the work of entities such as the "night hag" or "old hag," describing a malevolent presence that sits on the chest of sleeping individuals, causing feelings of pressure and suffocation.

2. Visits from Spirits or Ghosts:

- In some belief systems, sleep paralysis is interpreted as a form of spiritual visitation or communication with the spirit world.

- Individuals may report encounters with deceased loved ones, ancestral spirits, or otherworldly entities during sleep paralysis episodes, suggesting a connection to the afterlife or supernatural realms.

- These experiences are often deeply personal and may carry significant meaning or symbolism within the cultural and spiritual context of the individual.

3. Out-of-Body Experiences and Astral Projection:

- Some individuals who experience sleep paralysis report sensations of floating, levitating, or leaving their physical bodies during episodes.

- These experiences may be interpreted as instances of astral projection or out-of-body experiences, in which the consciousness or soul temporarily separates from the physical body and explores other dimensions or planes of existence.

- Proponents of astral projection suggest that sleep paralysis provides an opportunity for individuals to access higher realms of consciousness or spiritual enlightenment.

4. Interdimensional Phenomena:

- From a paranormal perspective, sleep paralysis may be seen as a window into other dimensions or alternate realities.

- Some theories propose that sleep paralysis allows individuals to perceive and interact with entities or beings from parallel universes, alternate timelines, or higher dimensions.

- These interpretations draw upon concepts from metaphysics, quantum physics, and fringe science to speculate on the nature of reality and the existence of unseen forces beyond conventional understanding.

5. Spiritual Awakening and Transformation:

- In certain spiritual traditions, sleep paralysis is viewed as a transformative experience that can lead to spiritual awakening, enlightenment, or personal growth.

- Individuals may interpret sleep paralysis episodes as initiatory or mystical encounters that facilitate spiritual development, inner healing, or expanded consciousness.

- These interpretations emphasize the potential for sleep paralysis to catalyze profound shifts in perception, belief, and identity, leading to greater self-awareness and spiritual evolution.

Overall, parapsychological and supernatural interpretations of sleep paralysis offer alternative perspectives on the phenomenon, inviting exploration of the mysteries of consciousness, spirituality, and the unknown. While these interpretations may not align with scientific explanations, they reflect the enduring fascination with the unexplained and the boundless possibilities of human experience.

6. Clinical Implications

- 6.1 Differential Diagnosis

Differential diagnosis involves distinguishing between sleep paralysis and other conditions that may present with similar symptoms or features. Here are some conditions that may be considered in the differential diagnosis of sleep paralysis:

1. Night Terrors and Nightmares:

- Night terrors and nightmares are sleep-related phenomena characterized by intense fear, distress, or arousal during sleep.

- Night terrors typically involve sudden awakening from sleep with extreme agitation, screaming, or thrashing, often accompanied by autonomic arousal.

- Nightmares are vivid and disturbing dreams that cause significant distress upon awakening, but they do not involve paralysis or muscle atonia.

2. Narcolepsy:

- Narcolepsy is a neurological disorder characterized by excessive daytime sleepiness, sudden loss of muscle tone (cataplexy), hallucinations, and disrupted sleep patterns.

- Sleep paralysis is a common symptom of narcolepsy and may occur as individuals transition between wakefulness and sleep, particularly during REM sleep.

3. Obstructive Sleep Apnea (OSA):

- Obstructive sleep apnea is a sleep disorder characterized by repetitive episodes of partial or complete obstruction of the upper airway during sleep, leading to pauses in breathing and disrupted sleep patterns.

- Individuals with OSA may experience episodes of arousal from sleep, gasping or choking sensations, and fragmented sleep architecture, but they typically do not experience paralysis during these episodes.

4. REM Sleep Behavior Disorder (RBD):

- REM sleep behavior disorder is a parasomnia characterized by the loss of normal muscle atonia during REM sleep, leading to the enactment of dream content through vocalizations, movements, or behaviors.

- Unlike sleep paralysis, which involves paralysis upon waking from sleep, RBD occurs during REM sleep and is associated with acting out dreams, often resulting in injury to oneself or bed partner.

5. Psychological Disorders:

- Psychological disorders such as panic disorder, anxiety disorders, and post-traumatic stress disorder (PTSD) may present with symptoms that overlap with sleep paralysis, including feelings of fear, panic, or dissociation.

- Differentiating between sleep paralysis and psychological disorders may involve assessing the timing, context, and associated features of the episodes, as well as conducting a comprehensive psychological evaluation.

6. Seizure Disorders:

- Certain seizure disorders, such as temporal lobe epilepsy, may present with symptoms that resemble sleep paralysis, including altered consciousness, sensory experiences, and motor phenomena.

- Differential diagnosis may involve conducting neuroimaging studies, electroencephalography (EEG), and other diagnostic tests to evaluate for underlying seizure activity or epilepsy.

7. Substance-Induced Sleep Disorders:

- Substance use, including alcohol, drugs, and medications, can disrupt sleep patterns and lead to experiences that resemble sleep paralysis.

- Differential diagnosis may involve assessing for substance use or medication side effects, as well as evaluating for other sleep-related disturbances or disorders.

8. Other Sleep Disorders:

- Other sleep disorders, such as periodic limb movement disorder (PLMD), restless legs syndrome (RLS), and circadian rhythm sleep-wake disorders, may present with symptoms that overlap with sleep paralysis.

- Differential diagnosis may involve considering the constellation of symptoms, sleep architecture findings, and associated features of these disorders.

Overall, conducting a thorough clinical evaluation, including a detailed history, physical examination, and diagnostic testing as needed, is essential for accurately diagnosing sleep paralysis and distinguishing it from other conditions with similar presentations. Collaboration between healthcare providers from multiple disciplines, including sleep medicine specialists, neurologists, psychiatrists, and psychologists, may be necessary to achieve an accurate differential diagnosis and develop an appropriate treatment plan.

- 6.2 Comorbidity with Other Sleep Disorders

Sleep paralysis can occur in conjunction with various other sleep disorders, either as a symptom of another underlying disorder or as a co-occurring condition. Here are some common comorbidities with sleep paralysis:

1. Narcolepsy:

   - Narcolepsy is a neurological disorder characterized by excessive daytime sleepiness, cataplexy (sudden loss of muscle tone), hallucinations, and disrupted nighttime sleep.

- Sleep paralysis is a frequent symptom of narcolepsy and often occurs during transitions between wakefulness and REM sleep, reflecting dysfunction in the regulation of sleep-wake cycles.

2. Obstructive Sleep Apnea (OSA):

- Obstructive sleep apnea is a sleep disorder characterized by repetitive episodes of partial or complete obstruction of the upper airway during sleep, leading to pauses in breathing and disrupted sleep patterns.

- Sleep paralysis may occur in individuals with OSA, particularly during episodes of hypnagogic (occurring while falling asleep) or hypnopompic (occurring while waking up) hallucinations associated with disrupted sleep architecture.

3. REM Sleep Behavior Disorder (RBD):

- REM sleep behavior disorder is a parasomnia characterized by the loss of normal muscle atonia during REM sleep, leading to the enactment of dream content through vocalizations, movements, or behaviors.

- While sleep paralysis involves paralysis upon waking from sleep, RBD occurs during REM sleep and is associated with acting out dreams, rather than experiencing paralysis.

4. Sleep-Related Anxiety Disorders:

- Anxiety disorders, such as panic disorder, generalized anxiety disorder (GAD), and post-traumatic stress disorder (PTSD), may co-occur with sleep paralysis and contribute to its frequency or severity.

- Individuals with sleep-related anxiety disorders may experience heightened arousal, fear, or panic during sleep paralysis episodes, leading to increased distress and impairment in sleep quality.

5. Insomnia:

- Insomnia involves difficulty falling asleep, staying asleep, or achieving restorative sleep, leading to daytime impairment and fatigue.

- Sleep paralysis may occur in individuals with insomnia, particularly during periods of fragmented sleep or sleep disturbances associated with anxiety or stress.

6. Restless Legs Syndrome (RLS) and Periodic Limb Movement Disorder (PLMD):

- RLS is characterized by uncomfortable sensations in the legs, often accompanied by an irresistible urge to move the legs to relieve discomfort, particularly at night.

- PLMD involves repetitive movements of the legs or arms during sleep, leading to disrupted sleep patterns and daytime fatigue.

- Sleep paralysis may co-occur with RLS or PLMD, although the mechanisms underlying this association are not fully understood.

7. Circadian Rhythm Sleep-Wake Disorders:

- Circadian rhythm sleep-wake disorders involve disruptions in the timing of sleep and wakefulness, leading to difficulties with sleep initiation, maintenance, or timing.

- Sleep paralysis may occur in individuals with circadian rhythm disorders, particularly during periods of sleep disruption or when the timing of REM sleep is altered.

Overall, identifying and addressing comorbid sleep disorders is essential for comprehensive management of sleep paralysis and improving overall sleep quality and daytime functioning. Treatment approaches may involve a combination of pharmacological interventions, cognitive-behavioral therapy (CBT), lifestyle modifications, and management of underlying medical or psychiatric conditions. Collaboration between healthcare providers from multiple disciplines, including sleep medicine specialists, neurologists, psychiatrists, and psychologists, may be necessary to address the complex interplay of sleep disorders and optimize treatment outcomes.

- 6.3 Impact on Mental Health

Sleep paralysis can have a significant impact on mental health, contributing to feelings of fear, anxiety, and distress, as well as disruptions in sleep quality and overall well-being. Here are some ways in which sleep paralysis can affect mental health:

1. Increased Anxiety and Fear:
   - Sleep paralysis episodes are often accompanied by intense feelings of fear, panic, or terror, particularly due to the

sensation of being unable to move or speak.

- Individuals may experience anticipatory anxiety or dread surrounding sleep, fearing the recurrence of sleep paralysis and its associated sensations.

- Chronic or recurrent sleep paralysis can exacerbate anxiety symptoms and contribute to overall psychological distress.

2. Disrupted Sleep Patterns:

- Sleep paralysis can disrupt the normal sleep-wake cycle and lead to fragmented sleep patterns, resulting in insufficient or poor-quality sleep.

- Sleep disturbances associated with sleep paralysis may contribute to daytime sleepiness, fatigue, and impaired cognitive function, impacting overall mental and physical health.

3. Negative Impact on Mood and Well-Being:

- The emotional toll of sleep paralysis, including feelings of helplessness, vulnerability, and dread, can negatively affect mood and overall well-being.

- Individuals may experience mood disturbances such as irritability, sadness, or decreased enjoyment of activities, particularly if sleep paralysis episodes occur frequently or are associated with distressing hallucinations.

4. Impaired Functioning and Performance:

- Sleep paralysis can impair daytime functioning and performance, leading to difficulties in concentration, memory, and productivity.

- Daytime sleepiness and fatigue resulting from disrupted sleep patterns may interfere with work, school, or social activities, contributing to functional impairment and decreased quality of life.

5. Psychological Symptoms and Disorders:

- Sleep paralysis may be associated with the development or exacerbation of psychological symptoms and disorders, including anxiety disorders, panic disorder, and post-traumatic stress disorder (PTSD).
- Individuals with pre-existing mental health conditions may be more vulnerable to the negative effects of sleep paralysis, and the presence of sleep disturbances can exacerbate psychiatric symptoms.

6. Impact on Daily Functioning and Relationships:

- The impact of sleep paralysis extends beyond individual well-being and may affect interpersonal relationships, social interactions, and daily functioning.
- Partners or family members may be unaware of the individual's experiences with sleep paralysis and may be unable

to provide support or understanding, leading to feelings of isolation or alienation.

Overall, sleep paralysis can have a profound impact on mental health, contributing to a range of psychological symptoms and impairments in daily functioning. Addressing sleep paralysis and its associated psychological effects may require a multifaceted approach, including education, coping strategies, psychological interventions, and, in some cases, pharmacological treatment. Seeking support from healthcare professionals, such as sleep specialists, psychologists, or psychiatrists, can help individuals manage the psychological impact of sleep paralysis and improve overall well-being.

- 6.4 Treatment and Management Options

Managing sleep paralysis involves addressing both the underlying factors contributing to the phenomenon and developing coping strategies to reduce the frequency and severity of episodes. Here are some treatment and management options for sleep paralysis:

1. Improving Sleep Hygiene:
- Establishing a regular sleep schedule and bedtime routine can help regulate the sleep-wake cycle and promote restful sleep.
- Creating a comfortable sleep environment free of distractions, noise, and excessive light can facilitate relaxation and improve sleep quality.

2. Stress Reduction Techniques:
- Practicing stress reduction techniques, such as mindfulness meditation, deep breathing exercises, or progressive muscle relaxation, can help alleviate anxiety and promote relaxation before bedtime.
- Engaging in activities that promote relaxation and stress relief, such as

yoga, tai chi, or listening to calming music, can also be beneficial.

3. Addressing Underlying Sleep Disorders:

- Treating underlying sleep disorders, such as narcolepsy, obstructive sleep apnea, or insomnia, may reduce the frequency or severity of sleep paralysis episodes.

- Consultation with a sleep specialist may be necessary to evaluate and diagnose any underlying sleep disorders and develop a targeted treatment plan.

4. Sleep Position and Environment Modification:

- Avoiding sleeping in supine (on the back) positions, which may increase the risk of sleep paralysis, and experimenting with alternative sleep positions may help reduce the occurrence of episodes.

- Making adjustments to the sleep environment, such as using supportive pillows, maintaining a comfortable room temperature, or using white noise machines, may also promote better sleep quality and reduce the likelihood of sleep paralysis.

5. Cognitive-Behavioral Therapy (CBT):

- Cognitive-behavioral therapy for insomnia (CBT-I) or for anxiety disorders (CBT-A) may be helpful in addressing maladaptive beliefs, thoughts, and behaviors associated with sleep paralysis.

- CBT techniques, such as cognitive restructuring, relaxation training, and sleep restriction therapy, can help individuals develop coping strategies and reduce the impact of sleep paralysis on mental health and well-being.

6. Medication:

- In some cases, medication may be prescribed to address underlying sleep disorders or to manage symptoms associated with sleep paralysis.

- Medications used to treat narcolepsy, such as stimulants (e.g., modafinil, methylphenidate) or sodium oxybate, may help improve symptoms of excessive daytime sleepiness and cataplexy associated with sleep paralysis in individuals with narcolepsy.

- However, medication should be used under the guidance of a healthcare professional and may not be appropriate for everyone.

7. Education and Support:

- Educating individuals about the nature of sleep paralysis, its prevalence, and potential contributing factors can help reduce fear and anxiety surrounding the phenomenon.

- Joining support groups or seeking support from healthcare professionals, therapists, or peer networks can provide validation, reassurance, and coping strategies for managing sleep paralysis.

8. Safety Precautions:

- Implementing safety precautions, such as removing obstacles or hazards from the sleep environment, can help prevent injuries during sleep paralysis episodes.

- Informing family members or bed partners about the individual's experiences with sleep paralysis and providing instructions for how to respond if assistance is needed can help alleviate concerns and ensure safety.

Overall, treatment and management of sleep paralysis involve a multidimensional approach that addresses both physiological and psychological factors contributing to the phenomenon. Tailoring interventions to individual needs and preferences can help individuals effectively manage sleep paralysis and improve overall sleep quality and well-being.

7. Coping Mechanisms and Prevention

- 7.1 Coping Strategies during Episodes

Coping strategies during sleep paralysis episodes can help individuals manage feelings of fear, anxiety, and helplessness, as well as reduce the duration and intensity of the experience. Here are some coping strategies that individuals can use during sleep paralysis episodes:

1. Stay Calm and Maintain Perspective:
 - Remind yourself that sleep paralysis is a temporary and usually harmless phenomenon.
 - Focus on staying calm and maintaining perspective, knowing that the episode will eventually pass.

2. Focus on Breathing:

- Focus on slow, deep breathing to promote relaxation and reduce feelings of anxiety.

- Concentrate on inhaling and exhaling slowly and steadily, using diaphragmatic breathing techniques if possible.

3. Attempt Small Movements:

- Try to initiate small movements, such as wiggling your fingers or toes, to signal to your brain that you are waking up.

- Gradually attempt to move larger muscle groups, such as your arms or legs, if possible.

4. Use Visualization Techniques:

- Visualize yourself in a peaceful and safe environment, such as a serene beach or calming nature scene.

- Use imagery to distract yourself from the sensations of paralysis and create a sense of relaxation and comfort.

5. Focus on Positive Thoughts:

- Redirect your thoughts toward positive and reassuring thoughts, such as affirmations or mantras.

- Repeat calming phrases or affirmations to yourself, such as "This will pass" or "I am safe and in control."

6. Attempt to Vocalize:

- Attempt to make vocal sounds, such as humming or whispering, to help stimulate muscle activity and signal to your brain that you are waking up.

- Focus on gradually regaining control over your vocal cords and speech muscles.

7. Use External Cues:

- If possible, try to focus on external sensory stimuli, such as the sound of a ticking clock or the feeling of your bed beneath you.

- Paying attention to external cues can help ground you in the present moment and reduce feelings of dissociation or disorientation.

8. Practice Acceptance and Mindfulness:

- Practice acceptance of the experience without judgment or resistance.

- Use mindfulness techniques to observe sensations, thoughts, and emotions without becoming overwhelmed by them.

9. Seek Support and Reassurance:

- If you feel comfortable, try to communicate with a bed partner or family member nearby to provide reassurance and support.

- Knowing that someone else is aware of your experience and available to assist you can help alleviate feelings of isolation and fear.

10. Follow Up with Healthcare Provider:

- If sleep paralysis episodes are frequent or causing significant distress, consider discussing them with a healthcare provider.

- A healthcare provider can provide further evaluation, offer support, and discuss potential treatment options if necessary.

It's important to remember that coping strategies may vary depending on individual preferences and experiences. Experiment with different techniques to find what works best for you, and don't hesitate to seek support from healthcare professionals or mental health providers if needed.

- 7.2 Lifestyle Changes for Prevention

Making lifestyle changes can help reduce the frequency and severity of sleep paralysis episodes. Here are some lifestyle changes that individuals can implement to prevent sleep paralysis:

1. Maintain a Regular Sleep Schedule:

- Establish a consistent sleep-wake schedule by going to bed and waking up at the same time every day, even on weekends.
- Consistency in sleep timing helps regulate the body's internal clock and promote healthy sleep patterns.

2. Create a Relaxing Bedtime Routine:

- Develop a calming bedtime routine to signal to your body that it's time to wind down and prepare for sleep.
- Engage in relaxing activities before bed, such as reading, taking a warm bath, or practicing relaxation techniques like deep breathing or meditation.

3. Optimize Sleep Environment:

- Create a comfortable and conducive sleep environment that promotes restful sleep.

- Keep your bedroom cool, dark, and quiet, and invest in a comfortable mattress and pillows to enhance sleep quality.

4. Practice Good Sleep Hygiene:

- Adopt healthy sleep habits to improve sleep quality and duration.

- Avoid caffeine, nicotine, and alcohol close to bedtime, as they can disrupt sleep patterns and contribute to sleep disturbances.

5. Manage Stress and Anxiety:

- Implement stress-reduction techniques to manage anxiety and promote relaxation.

- Practice mindfulness meditation, yoga, or progressive muscle relaxation to reduce stress levels and promote better sleep.

6. Avoid Sleep Deprivation:

- Prioritize getting an adequate amount of sleep each night to prevent sleep deprivation.

- Aim for 7-9 hours of quality sleep per night, as insufficient sleep can increase the likelihood of experiencing sleep paralysis episodes.

7. Address Underlying Health Conditions:

- Manage underlying health conditions that may contribute to sleep disturbances or exacerbate sleep paralysis.

- Seek treatment for conditions such as sleep apnea, restless legs syndrome, or mental health disorders that may affect sleep quality.

8. Limit Screen Time Before Bed:

- Minimize exposure to electronic devices, such as smartphones, computers, and televisions, before bedtime.

- Blue light emitted by screens can disrupt the production of melatonin, a hormone that regulates sleep-wake cycles, so it's best to avoid screens at least an hour before bed.

9. Exercise Regularly:

- Engage in regular physical activity, but avoid vigorous exercise close to bedtime.

- Regular exercise can promote better sleep quality and reduce stress, anxiety, and symptoms of depression that may contribute to sleep paralysis.

10. Seek Support and Education:

- Educate yourself about sleep paralysis and its triggers to better understand your experiences and develop coping strategies.

- Seek support from healthcare providers, sleep specialists, or support groups to address any concerns or questions you may have about sleep paralysis.

By incorporating these lifestyle changes into your daily routine, you can create a healthier sleep environment and reduce the likelihood of experiencing sleep paralysis episodes. Experiment with different strategies to find what works best for you, and remember to be patient and consistent in your efforts to improve sleep quality and overall well-being.

- 7.3 Psychological Interventions

Psychological interventions can be effective in managing sleep paralysis by addressing underlying psychological factors, reducing anxiety, and improving coping strategies. Here are some psychological interventions that may be helpful:

1. Cognitive-Behavioral Therapy (CBT):

- CBT is a structured, evidence-based therapy that focuses on identifying and changing negative thought patterns and behaviors associated with sleep paralysis.

- In CBT for sleep paralysis, individuals learn to recognize and challenge irrational beliefs and fears about sleep paralysis, develop relaxation techniques to reduce anxiety, and implement behavioral strategies to improve sleep hygiene.

2. Exposure Therapy:

- Exposure therapy involves gradually exposing individuals to feared situations or stimuli associated with sleep paralysis in a controlled and systematic manner.

- Through repeated exposure to sleep paralysis-related triggers, individuals can learn to habituate to the experience, reduce avoidance behaviors, and decrease anxiety over time.

3. Mindfulness-Based Interventions:

- Mindfulness-based interventions, such as mindfulness meditation and mindfulness-based stress reduction (MBSR), teach individuals to cultivate present-moment awareness and nonjudgmental acceptance of thoughts, emotions, and sensations.

- Mindfulness practices can help individuals develop greater resilience to distressing experiences like sleep paralysis, reduce reactivity to intrusive thoughts or sensations, and promote relaxation and emotional well-being.

4. Imagery Rehearsal Therapy (IRT):

- IRT involves using visualization and imagery techniques to rehearse positive and adaptive responses to sleep paralysis episodes.

- Individuals practice imagining themselves successfully coping with sleep paralysis, visualizing themselves remaining calm, moving freely, and feeling safe during episodes.

5. Relaxation Techniques:

- Various relaxation techniques, such as progressive muscle relaxation, deep breathing exercises, and guided imagery, can help individuals manage anxiety and promote relaxation before bedtime.

- Practicing relaxation techniques regularly can reduce physiological arousal, improve sleep quality, and decrease the likelihood of experiencing sleep paralysis episodes.

6. Stress Management Skills:

- Learning stress management skills, such as problem-solving, time management, and assertiveness training, can help individuals address sources of stress and build resilience to sleep disturbances.

- Identifying and addressing stressors in daily life can reduce overall anxiety levels and create a more conducive environment for restful sleep.

7. Coping Skills Training:

-   Coping skills training teaches individuals adaptive strategies for managing distressing emotions and challenging situations.

- Individuals learn techniques such as cognitive restructuring, emotion regulation, and problem-solving to cope effectively with sleep paralysis episodes and associated anxiety.

8. Psychoeducation:

- Providing education about sleep paralysis, its prevalence, and potential contributing factors can help individuals develop a greater understanding of their experiences and reduce fear and misconceptions.

-   Psychoeducation can empower individuals to take an active role in managing sleep paralysis and seeking appropriate support and resources.

These psychological interventions can be delivered individually or in group settings, depending on the individual's preferences and needs. Working with a trained therapist or mental health professional can help individuals tailor interventions to their specific circumstances and develop personalized strategies for managing sleep paralysis effectively.

8. Future Directions and Research

- 8.1 Advances in Sleep Science

Recent advances in sleep science have led to a deeper understanding of the mechanisms underlying sleep paralysis and its associated phenomena. Here are some notable advances in sleep science related to sleep paralysis:

1. Neurobiological Mechanisms:

-      Advances in neuroimaging techniques, such as functional magnetic resonance imaging (fMRI) and positron emission tomography (PET), have allowed researchers to investigate the neural correlates of sleep paralysis.

- Studies have identified alterations in brain activity and connectivity during sleep paralysis episodes, particularly involving regions of the brain responsible for motor control, sensory processing, and self-awareness.

2. Genetic and Familial Factors:

- Research has explored genetic and familial factors contributing to sleep paralysis susceptibility and its association with other sleep disorders, such as narcolepsy.

- Genome-wide association studies (GWAS) and genetic linkage analyses have identified potential genetic variants and heritable traits associated with sleep paralysis, shedding light on its underlying genetic architecture.

3. REM Sleep Dysregulation:

- Advances in understanding the regulation of rapid eye movement (REM) sleep have provided insights into the mechanisms underlying sleep paralysis.

- Dysregulation of REM sleep, including abnormalities in REM sleep onset, duration, and muscle atonia, has been implicated in the pathophysiology of sleep paralysis and its associated phenomena.

4. Psychological and Cognitive Factors:

- Research has focused on the role of psychological and cognitive factors in shaping individuals' experiences of sleep paralysis and their interpretations of the phenomenon.
- Studies have investigated the influence of stress, anxiety, trauma, cultural beliefs, and cognitive biases on the occurrence and perception of sleep paralysis episodes, highlighting the complex interplay of psychological factors in shaping subjective experiences.

5. Virtual Reality and Simulation Studies:

- Virtual reality (VR) technology and simulation studies have been used to recreate and study sleep paralysis experiences in controlled laboratory settings.
- VR-based experiments allow researchers to manipulate sensory

inputs, induce sleep paralysis-like states, and investigate the impact of environmental factors on the subjective experience of sleep paralysis.

6. Treatment Approaches:

- Advances in treatment approaches for sleep paralysis have included the development of targeted interventions, such as cognitive-behavioral therapy (CBT) and exposure therapy.

- Research has evaluated the efficacy of psychological interventions, pharmacological treatments, and lifestyle modifications in reducing the frequency and severity of sleep paralysis episodes and improving overall sleep quality and well-being.

7. Cross-Disciplinary Collaboration:

- Collaboration between sleep scientists, neuroscientists, psychologists, psychiatrists, and other disciplines has facilitated a multidimensional understanding of sleep paralysis and its implications for mental health, consciousness, and human experience.

- Integrating insights from diverse fields has enriched our understanding of sleep paralysis as a complex and multifaceted phenomenon with biological, psychological, and cultural dimensions.

Overall, recent advances in sleep science have expanded our knowledge of sleep paralysis and provided new avenues for research, diagnosis, and treatment. Continued interdisciplinary collaboration and innovative research approaches are essential for further unraveling the mysteries of sleep paralysis and its impact on sleep health and human consciousness.

Emerging research and innovative approaches have led to the exploration of novel therapeutic strategies for managing sleep paralysis. While there isn't a specific medication approved solely for treating sleep paralysis, various interventions may help alleviate symptoms and improve overall sleep quality. Here are some novel therapeutic approaches being investigated:

1. Pharmacological Interventions:
- Although no medications are currently approved specifically for sleep paralysis, certain pharmacological agents used to treat related sleep disorders may be beneficial. For example, sodium oxybate, which is commonly used to manage symptoms of narcolepsy, has been studied for its potential efficacy in reducing sleep paralysis episodes.

- Other medications, such as selective serotonin reuptake inhibitors (SSRIs) or tricyclic antidepressants, which are commonly used to treat anxiety and depression, may also be considered in individuals with sleep paralysis associated with psychological distress.

2. Targeted Neurotransmitter Modulation:

- Research is exploring the role of neurotransmitters, such as serotonin, dopamine, and gamma-aminobutyric acid (GABA), in the regulation of sleep-wake cycles and REM sleep. Modulating these neurotransmitter systems through targeted pharmacological interventions may offer novel approaches for managing sleep paralysis.

- Investigational agents targeting specific neurotransmitter receptors or pathways involved in REM sleep regulation are being explored for their potential to modulate sleep paralysis episodes.

3. Neuromodulation Techniques:

-    Non-invasive neuromodulation techniques, such as transcranial magnetic stimulation (TMS) or transcranial direct current stimulation (tDCS), are being investigated as potential treatments for sleep disorders, including sleep paralysis.

-    These techniques involve the application of electromagnetic fields or electrical currents to specific regions of the brain to modulate neural activity and promote changes in sleep architecture.

4. Virtual Reality Therapy:

- Virtual reality (VR) therapy involves exposing individuals to simulated environments or scenarios to evoke specific sensations or experiences.

- VR-based interventions for sleep paralysis may include exposure therapy, where individuals are gradually exposed to virtual representations of sleep paralysis-related stimuli in a controlled and therapeutic setting to reduce fear and anxiety associated with the experience.

5. Mind-Body Interventions:

- Mind-body interventions, such as biofeedback, mindfulness meditation, and yoga, are being explored as adjunctive therapies for managing sleep paralysis and associated psychological symptoms.

- These practices promote self-awareness, relaxation, and stress reduction, which may help individuals cope with sleep paralysis episodes and improve overall sleep quality.

6. Gene Therapy and Genetic Targeting:

- Advances in genetic research have identified potential genetic factors associated with sleep paralysis susceptibility and REM sleep dysregulation.

- Gene therapy approaches targeting specific genetic variants or pathways implicated in sleep paralysis may offer future therapeutic options for individuals with severe or refractory cases of the disorder.

7. Behavioral and Lifestyle Interventions:

- Lifestyle modifications, such as optimizing sleep hygiene, managing stress, and promoting relaxation before bedtime, remain essential components of sleep paralysis management.

- Behavioral interventions, including cognitive-behavioral therapy (CBT) and exposure therapy, continue to be investigated for their efficacy in reducing the frequency and severity of sleep paralysis episodes and improving overall sleep quality and well-being.

While these novel therapeutic approaches hold promise for the future management of sleep paralysis, further research is needed to evaluate their safety, efficacy, and long-term outcomes. Collaborative efforts between researchers, clinicians, and industry partners are essential for advancing our understanding of sleep paralysis and developing effective treatments that address the complex interplay of biological, psychological, and environmental factors involved in the disorder.

- 8.3 Unanswered Questions and Areas for Further Study

Despite advancements in sleep science and the exploration of therapeutic interventions, several unanswered questions and areas for further study remain regarding sleep paralysis. Here are some key questions and topics that warrant continued investigation:

1. Underlying Mechanisms:

- What specific neurobiological mechanisms contribute to the occurrence of sleep paralysis episodes?

- How do alterations in REM sleep regulation, neurotransmitter function, and brain connectivity influence the pathophysiology of sleep paralysis?

2. Genetic and Familial Factors:

- What genetic variants and heritable traits are associated with susceptibility to sleep paralysis?

- Are there specific genetic markers or familial patterns that predispose individuals to experiencing sleep paralysis?

3. Psychological and Cultural Factors:

- How do psychological factors, such as stress, anxiety, trauma, and cultural beliefs, shape individuals' experiences of sleep paralysis?

- What cultural variations exist in the prevalence, interpretation, and management of sleep paralysis across different populations and societies?

4. Impact on Mental Health:

- What are the long-term psychological consequences of recurrent sleep paralysis episodes?

- How does sleep paralysis contribute to the development or exacerbation of mental health disorders, such as anxiety, depression, and post-traumatic stress disorder (PTSD)?

5. Treatment Efficacy and Optimization:

- What are the most effective treatment approaches for managing sleep paralysis, both pharmacological and non-pharmacological?

- How can existing therapeutic interventions be optimized to better address the diverse needs and preferences of individuals with sleep paralysis?

6. Risk Factors and Predictors:

- What demographic, clinical, and environmental factors increase the risk of experiencing sleep paralysis?

- Are there specific predictors or early warning signs that can identify individuals at higher risk for developing sleep paralysis?

7. Comorbidity with Other Sleep Disorders:

- What are the prevalence and clinical implications of comorbid sleep disorders, such as narcolepsy, insomnia, and obstructive sleep apnea, in individuals with sleep paralysis?

- How do comorbid sleep disorders influence the presentation, course, and treatment response of sleep paralysis?

8. Cross-Cultural Variations:

- How do cultural beliefs, folklore, and mythological narratives influence the interpretation and experience of sleep paralysis across different cultural contexts?

- Are there cultural-specific interventions or approaches for managing sleep paralysis that warrant further investigation?

9. Impact on Quality of Life:

- What is the overall impact of sleep paralysis on individuals' quality of life, functioning, and well-being?

- How does the frequency, severity, and duration of sleep paralysis episodes affect individuals' daily functioning, relationships, and occupational performance?

10. Ethical and Legal Considerations:

- What ethical considerations arise in the diagnosis, treatment, and research of sleep paralysis, particularly concerning informed consent, privacy, and patient autonomy?

- What are the legal implications of sleep paralysis-related phenomena, such as sleep-related accidents or injuries, and how can they be addressed within healthcare and legal frameworks?

Addressing these unanswered questions and areas for further study will require interdisciplinary collaboration, rigorous research methodologies, and engagement with diverse populations to advance our understanding of sleep paralysis and improve clinical care and outcomes for affected individuals.

9. <u>Conclusion</u>

- 9.1 Recapitulation of Key Points

1. Definition and Characteristics:
- Sleep paralysis is a phenomenon characterized by temporary muscle paralysis occurring during transitions between sleep and wakefulness, often accompanied by hallucinations and a sense of fear or dread.
- It typically occurs during rapid eye movement (REM) sleep or upon awakening from REM sleep.

2. Prevalence and Occurrence:
- Sleep paralysis is relatively common, with prevalence rates varying across populations and studies.
- It can occur in individuals of any age, but it is more common in adolescents and young adults.

- Sleep paralysis is often associated with REM sleep, during which dreaming occurs and muscle atonia is present to prevent acting out dreams.

- It can also occur during the transition between wakefulness and sleep (hypnagogic) or between sleep and wakefulness (hypnopompic).

4. REM Sleep and Muscle Atonia:

- REM sleep is characterized by rapid eye movements, vivid dreaming, and muscle atonia, which is the temporary paralysis of skeletal muscles.

- Muscle atonia during REM sleep is believed to be mediated by inhibitory signals from the brainstem, preventing individuals from physically acting out their dreams.

5. Understanding Sleep Paralysis:

- Sleep paralysis results from a disruption in the normal transition between sleep stages, leading to a dissociation between consciousness and muscle control.

- Episodes are often accompanied by hallucinations, sensory experiences, and intense emotions.

6. Types of Sleep Paralysis:

- Sleep paralysis can be categorized into isolated sleep paralysis, occurring sporadically, and recurrent isolated sleep paralysis, involving frequent episodes over time.

- It may also occur as part of other sleep disorders, such as narcolepsy with cataplexy.

7. Symptoms and Experiences:

- Common symptoms of sleep paralysis include the inability to move or speak, sensations of pressure or suffocation, visual or auditory hallucinations, and feelings of fear or impending doom.

- Experiences during sleep paralysis episodes can vary widely among individuals and cultures.

8. Factors Contributing to Sleep Paralysis:

- Various factors may contribute to the occurrence of sleep paralysis, including sleep deprivation, irregular sleep schedules, stress, anxiety, and certain sleep disorders.

- Genetic and familial factors may also play a role in susceptibility to sleep paralysis.

9. Impact on Mental Health:

- Sleep paralysis can have a significant impact on mental health, leading to feelings of fear, anxiety, and distress, as well as disruptions in sleep quality and overall well-being.

- It may be associated with the development or exacerbation of psychological symptoms and disorders, such as anxiety disorders and post-traumatic stress disorder (PTSD).

10. Treatment and Management Options:

- Management of sleep paralysis involves addressing underlying factors contributing to the phenomenon and developing coping strategies to reduce the frequency and severity of episodes.

- Treatment options may include improving sleep hygiene, managing stress and anxiety, seeking support from healthcare professionals, and considering pharmacological interventions or psychological therapies.

These key points provide a comprehensive overview of sleep paralysis, its characteristics, contributing factors, impact on mental health, and approaches to treatment and management. Further research and understanding of sleep paralysis are essential for improving diagnosis, treatment, and support for individuals affected by this phenomenon.

- 9.2 Implications for Clinical Practice and Public Health

The understanding of sleep paralysis has several implications for clinical practice and public health:

1. Clinical Assessment and Diagnosis:

- Healthcare providers should be aware of the characteristics and diagnostic criteria for sleep paralysis to accurately identify and assess individuals experiencing this phenomenon.

- Comprehensive clinical evaluations, including detailed sleep histories, physical examinations, and sleep studies, may be necessary to differentiate sleep paralysis from other sleep disorders and medical conditions.

2. Treatment and Management Strategies:

- Healthcare professionals should be knowledgeable about the range of treatment and management options available for sleep paralysis, including lifestyle modifications, psychological interventions, and pharmacological therapies.

- Individualized treatment plans should be tailored to address the specific needs, preferences, and underlying factors contributing to sleep paralysis in each patient.

3. Psychoeducation and Support:

- Psychoeducation about sleep paralysis, its prevalence, and potential contributing factors can help alleviate fear, anxiety, and misconceptions surrounding the phenomenon.

- Providing support and reassurance to individuals experiencing sleep paralysis can promote a sense of validation, reduce feelings of isolation, and empower individuals to seek appropriate care and resources.

4. Screening for Comorbidities:

- Healthcare providers should screen individuals with sleep paralysis for comorbid sleep disorders, mental health conditions, and other medical comorbidities that may impact treatment outcomes and overall well-being.

- Integrated care approaches may be beneficial for addressing the complex interplay of physical, psychological, and social factors associated with sleep paralysis.

5. Public Health Awareness and Education:

- Public health campaigns and educational initiatives can raise awareness about sleep paralysis and its prevalence, symptoms, and potential impact on mental health.

- Targeted outreach efforts may be needed to reach underserved populations, promote early recognition of sleep paralysis symptoms, and encourage help-seeking behaviors among affected individuals.

6. Research and Innovation:

- Continued research into the underlying mechanisms, risk factors, and treatment approaches for sleep paralysis is essential for advancing clinical practice and public health initiatives.

- Collaborative efforts between researchers, healthcare providers, policymakers, and community stakeholders can facilitate knowledge translation and the implementation of evidence-based practices in clinical settings.

By integrating knowledge about sleep paralysis into clinical practice and public health efforts, healthcare providers and policymakers can improve the recognition, diagnosis, treatment, and support for individuals affected by this phenomenon. By addressing the physical, psychological, and social dimensions of sleep paralysis, healthcare systems can enhance the quality of care and promote better sleep health outcomes for affected individuals.

- 9.3 Final Thoughts and Considerations

In conclusion, sleep paralysis is a fascinating yet often distressing phenomenon that occurs during transitions between sleep and wakefulness. It is characterized by temporary muscle paralysis, often accompanied by hallucinations and a sense of fear or dread. While sleep paralysis is relatively common and usually harmless, it can have significant implications for mental health and well-being, particularly when accompanied by intense anxiety or distress.

Understanding sleep paralysis requires a multidimensional approach that considers biological, psychological, and cultural factors. Healthcare providers play a crucial role in recognizing and assessing sleep paralysis, providing education and support to affected individuals, and implementing evidence-based treatment and management strategies. Public health initiatives aimed at raising awareness, promoting early recognition, and reducing stigma surrounding sleep paralysis can further support affected individuals and improve access to care.

As research into sleep paralysis continues to evolve, it is important to prioritize the voices and experiences of individuals affected by this phenomenon. By listening to their perspectives, addressing their concerns, and advocating for their needs, healthcare providers and policymakers can foster a more compassionate and inclusive approach to sleep health.

Ultimately, by working collaboratively across disciplines and communities, we can enhance our understanding of sleep paralysis, improve clinical care and support, and promote better sleep health outcomes for all.

www.ingramcontent.com/pod-product-compliance
Lightning Source LLC
Chambersburg PA
CBHW061053250726
48653CB00001B/385